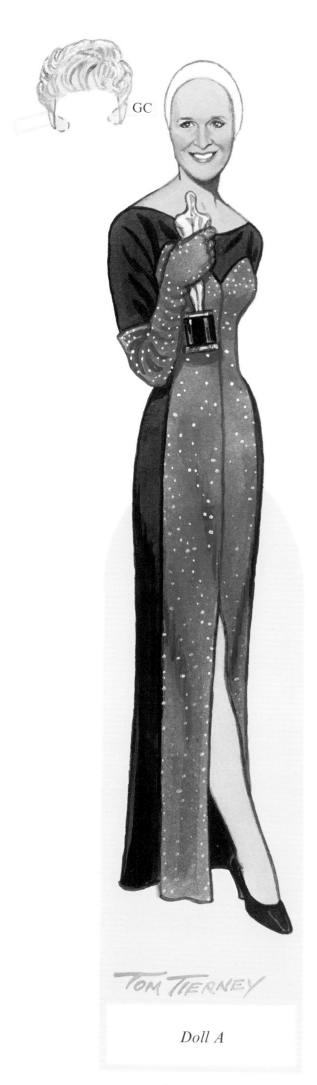

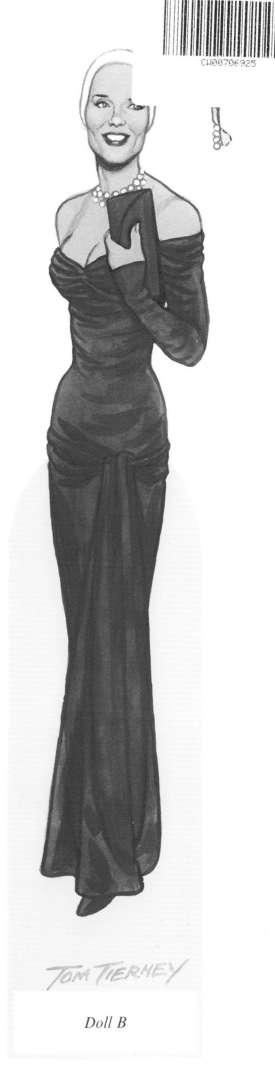

Doll A

Glenn Close
Academy Awards 1990

Doll B

Geena Davis
Academy Awards 1990

PLATE 1

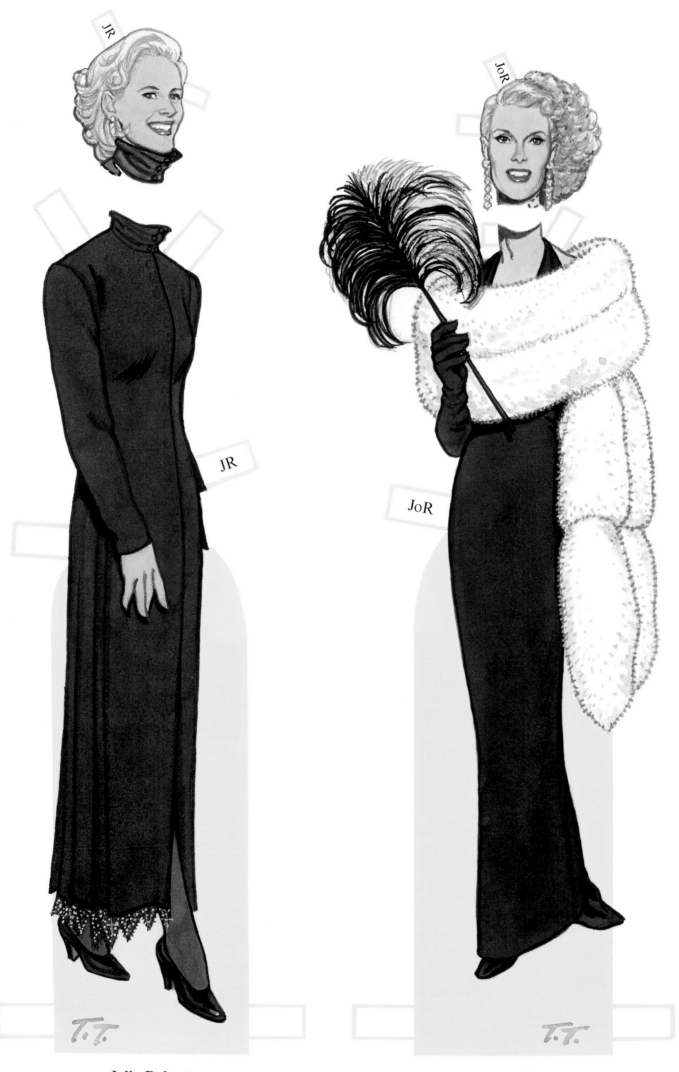

Julia Roberts
Academy Awards 1991

Joan Rivers
Black-and-White Fundraiser 1991

PLATE 2

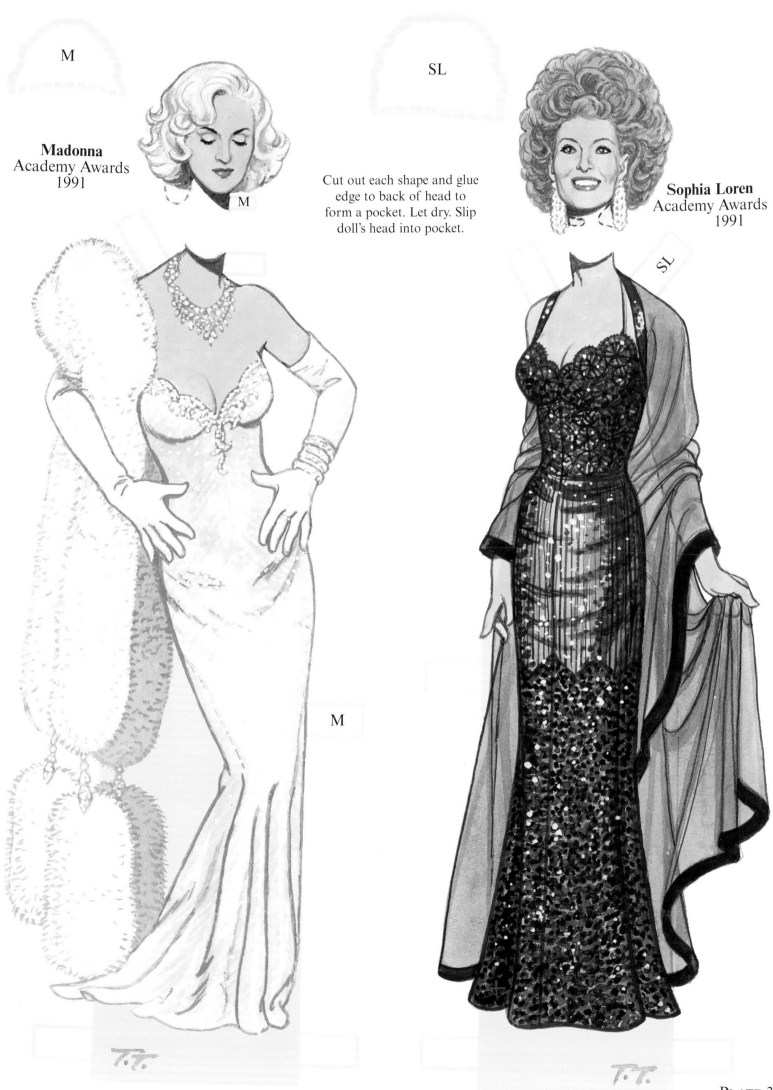

M

Madonna
Academy Awards
1991

M

Cut out each shape and glue
edge to back of head to
form a pocket. Let dry. Slip
doll's head into pocket.

SL

Sophia Loren
Academy Awards
1991

SL

M

PLATE 3

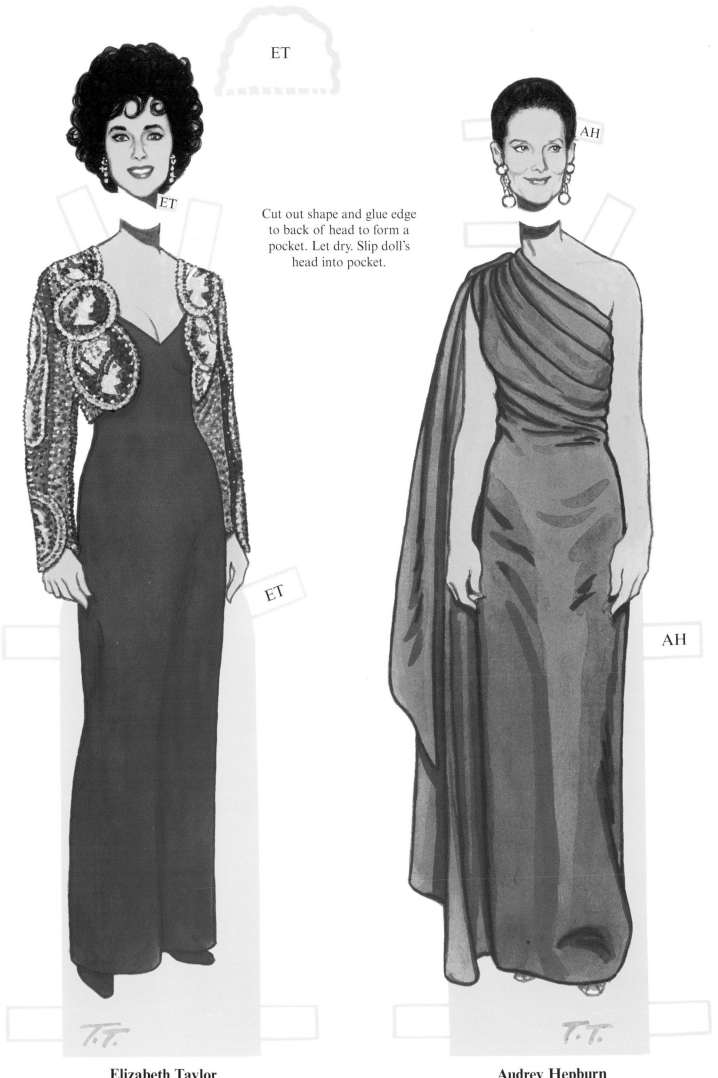

ET

Cut out shape and glue edge to back of head to form a pocket. Let dry. Slip doll's head into pocket.

ET

AH

ET

AH

Elizabeth Taylor
AIDS Benefit 1992

Audrey Hepburn
Academy Awards 1992

PLATE 4

Demi Moore
Academy Awards 1992

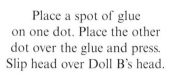

Place a spot of glue
on one dot. Place the other
dot over the glue and press.
Slip head over Doll B's head.

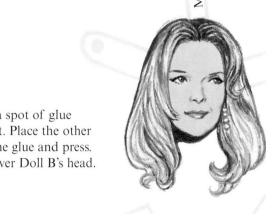

Michelle Pfeiffer
Golden Globes 1993

Do not cut out
space between
arm and body.

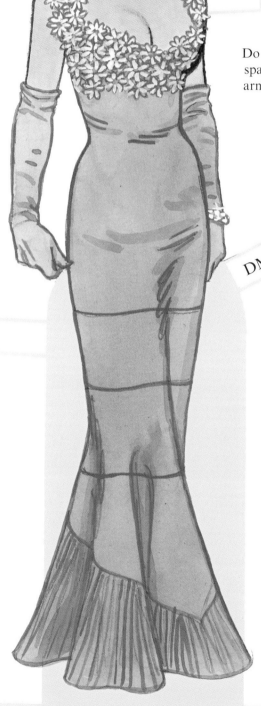

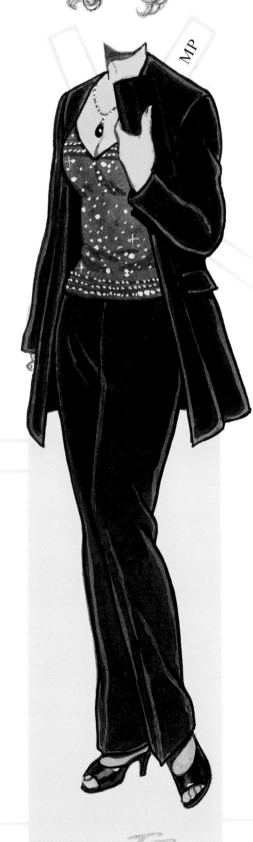

PLATE 5

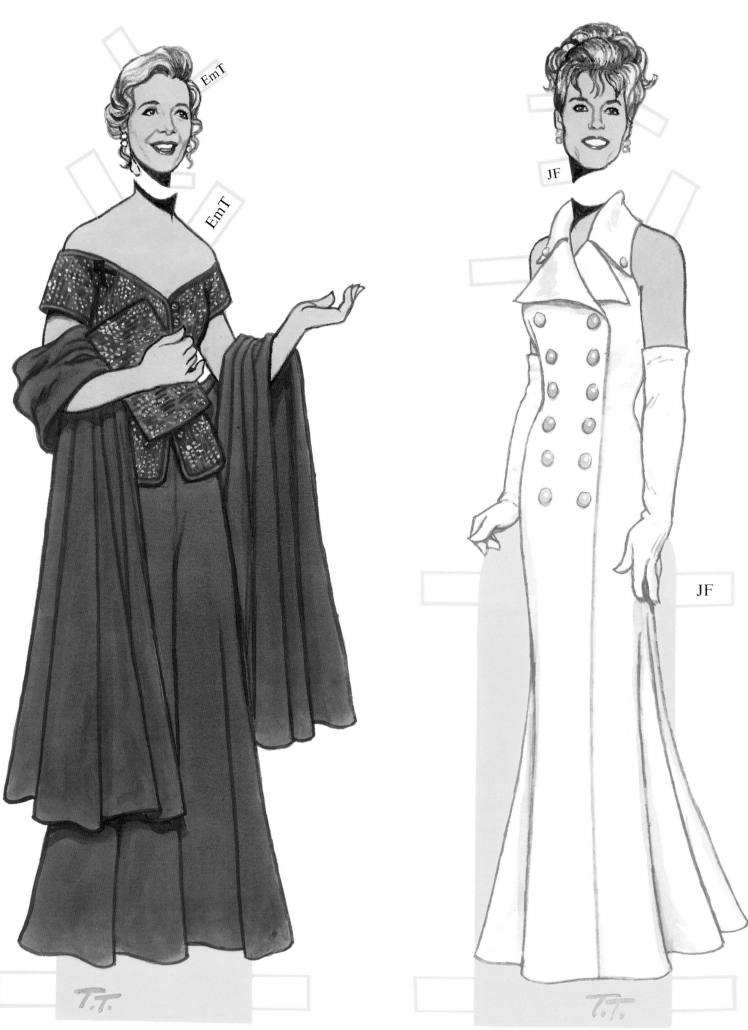

Emma Thompson
Academy Awards 1993

PLATE 6

Jane Fonda
Academy Awards 1993

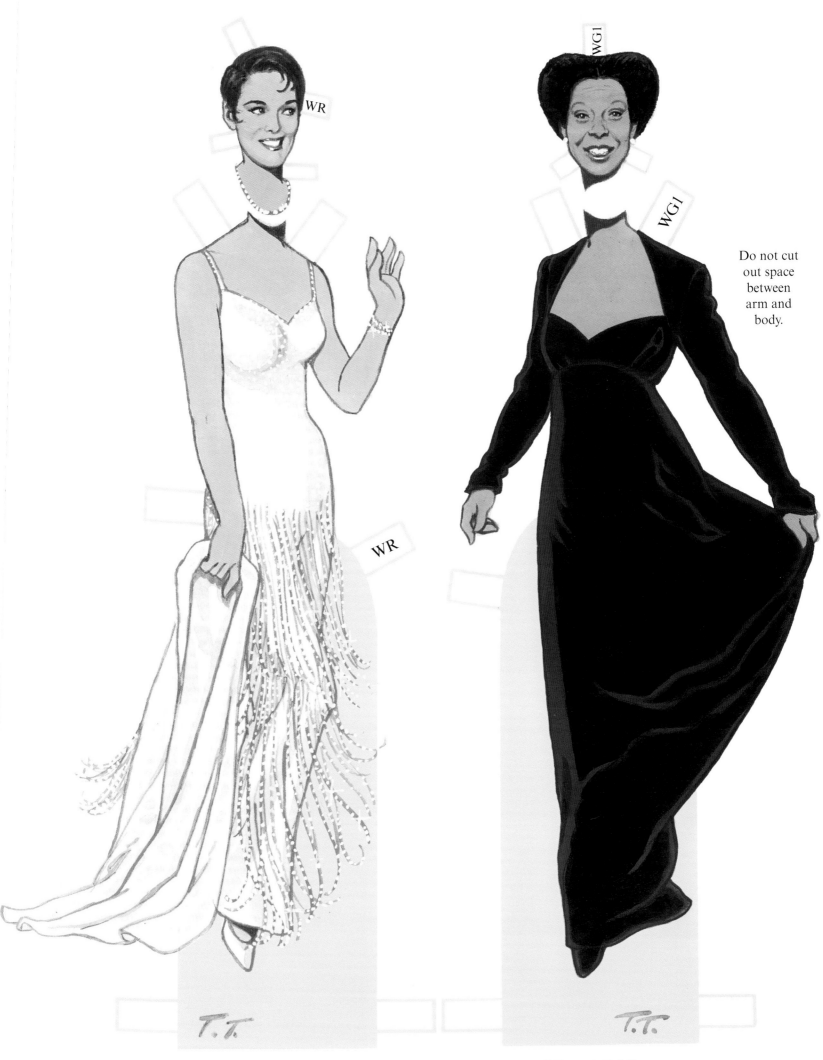

Do not cut out space between arm and body.

Winona Ryder
Academy Awards 1994

Whoopi Goldberg
Academy Awards 1994

PLATE 7

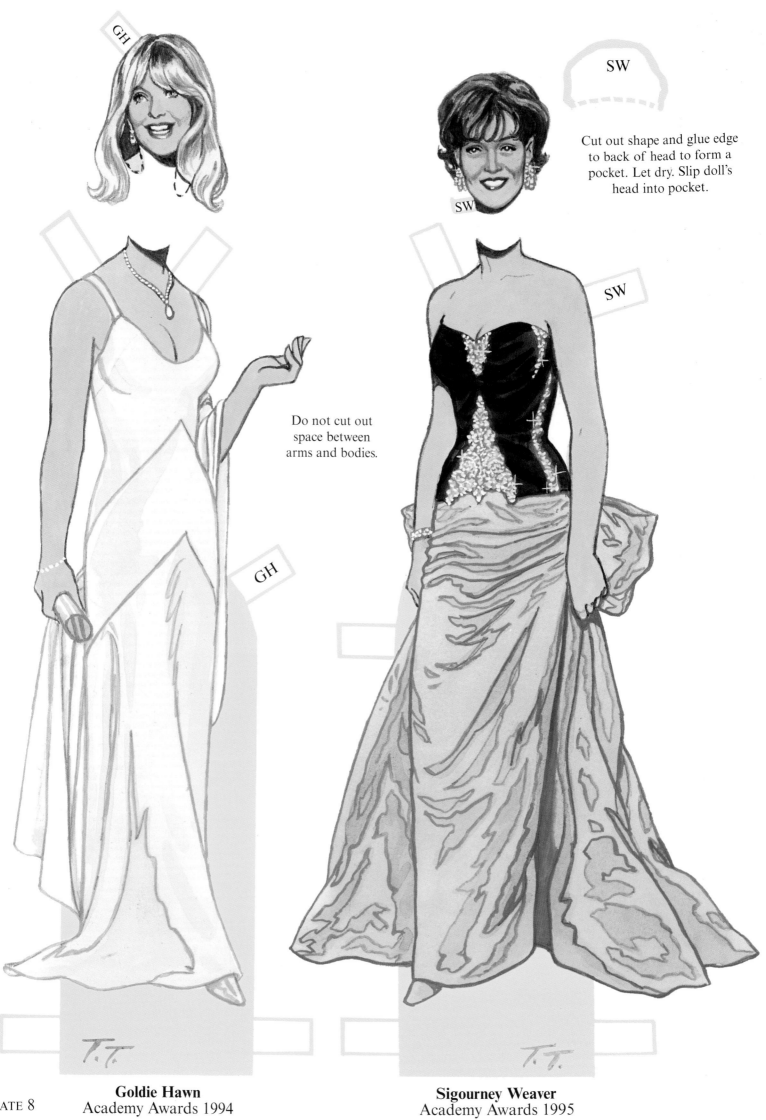

GH

SW

Cut out shape and glue edge to back of head to form a pocket. Let dry. Slip doll's head into pocket.

SW

Do not cut out space between arms and bodies.

SW

GH

Goldie Hawn
Academy Awards 1994

Sigourney Weaver
Academy Awards 1995

PLATE 8

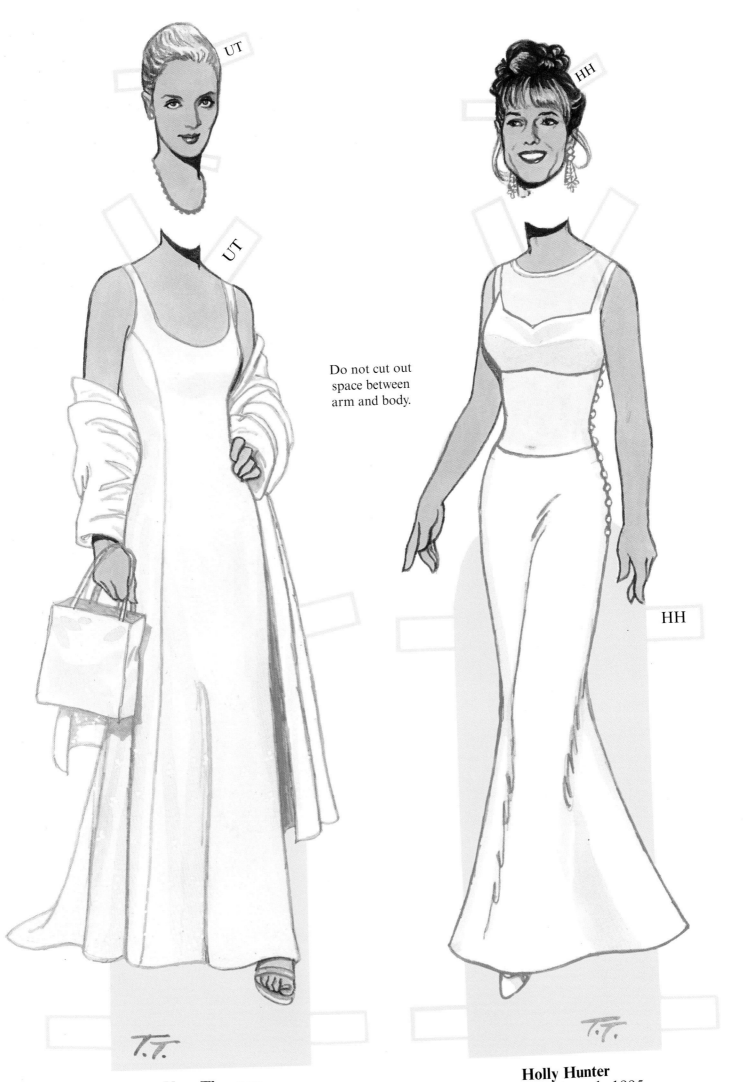

Do not cut out space between arm and body.

UT

UT

HH

HH

Uma Thurman
Academy Awards 1995

Holly Hunter
Academy Awards 1995

PLATE 9

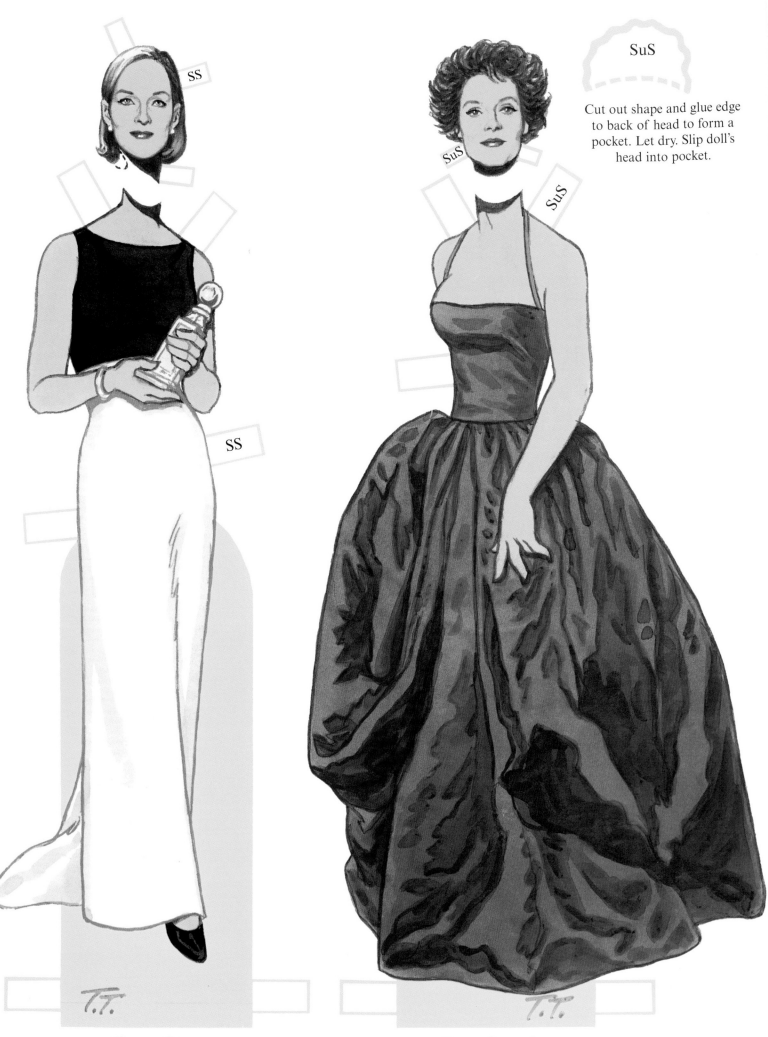

SS

SS

SuS

SuS

SuS

Cut out shape and glue edge to back of head to form a pocket. Let dry. Slip doll's head into pocket.

Sharon Stone
Golden Globes 1996

Susan Sarandon
Academy Awards 1996

PLATE 10

Sandra Bullock
Academy Awards 1996

Nicole Kidman
Academy Awards 1997

NK

SB

Do not cut out
space between
arms and bodies.

SB

NK

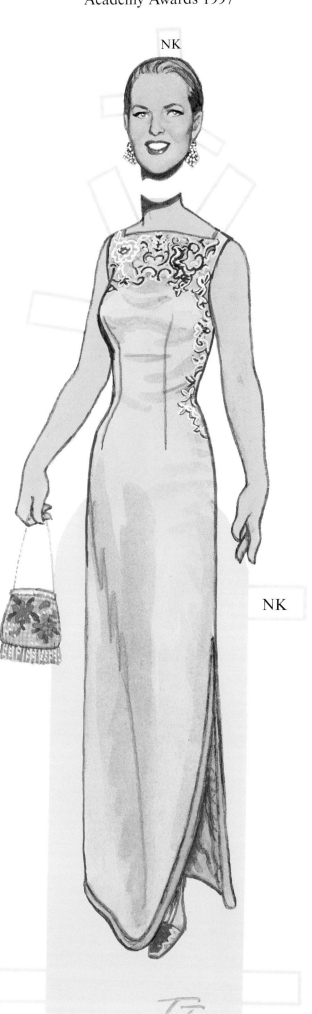

PLATE 11

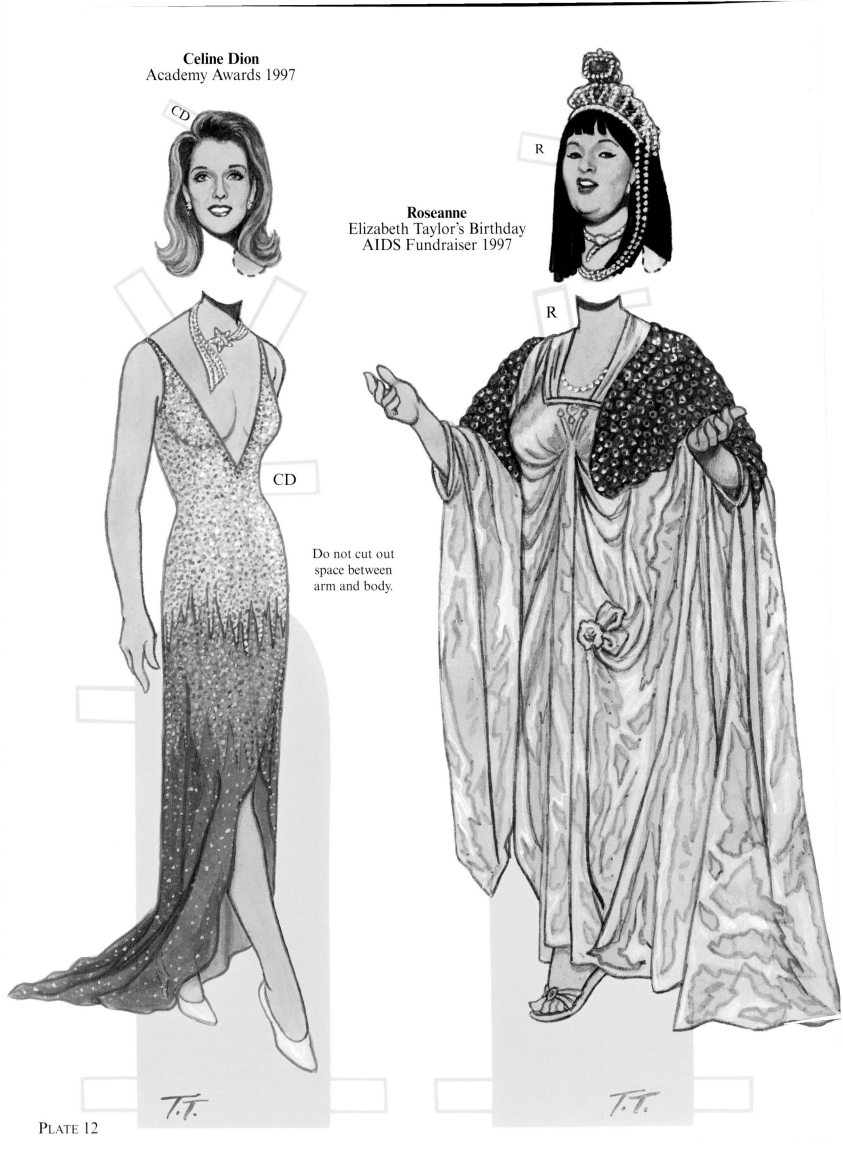

Celine Dion
Academy Awards 1997

CD

CD

Do not cut out
space between
arm and body.

Roseanne
Elizabeth Taylor's Birthday
AIDS Fundraiser 1997

R

R

T.T.

T.T.

PLATE 12

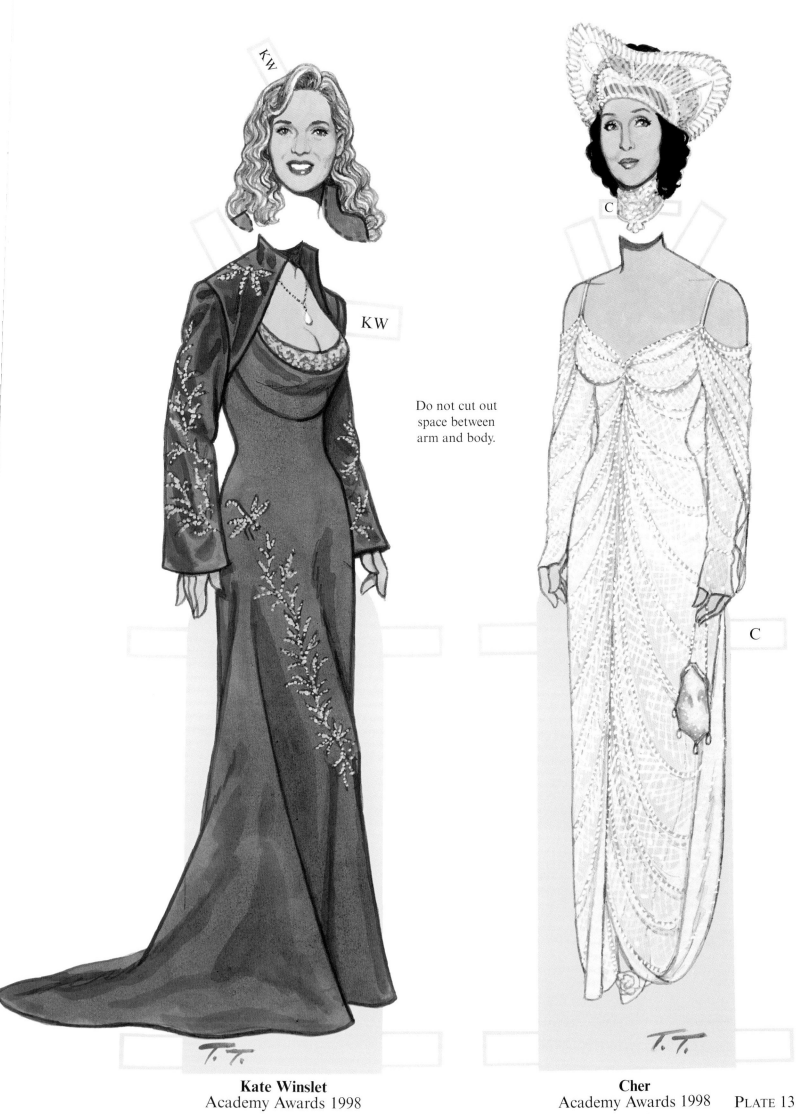

Do not cut out space between arm and body.

Kate Winslet
Academy Awards 1998

Cher
Academy Awards 1998 PLATE 13

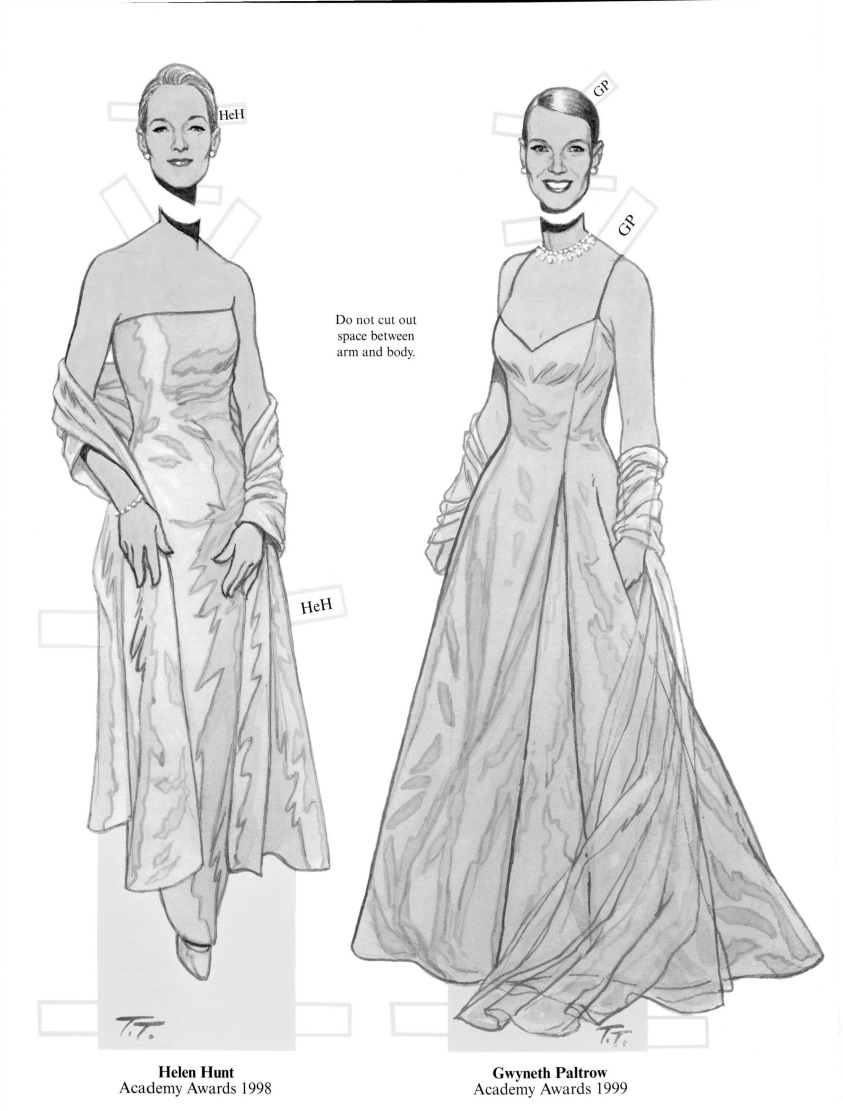

Do not cut out
space between
arm and body.

Helen Hunt
Academy Awards 1998

Gwyneth Paltrow
Academy Awards 1999

PLATE 14

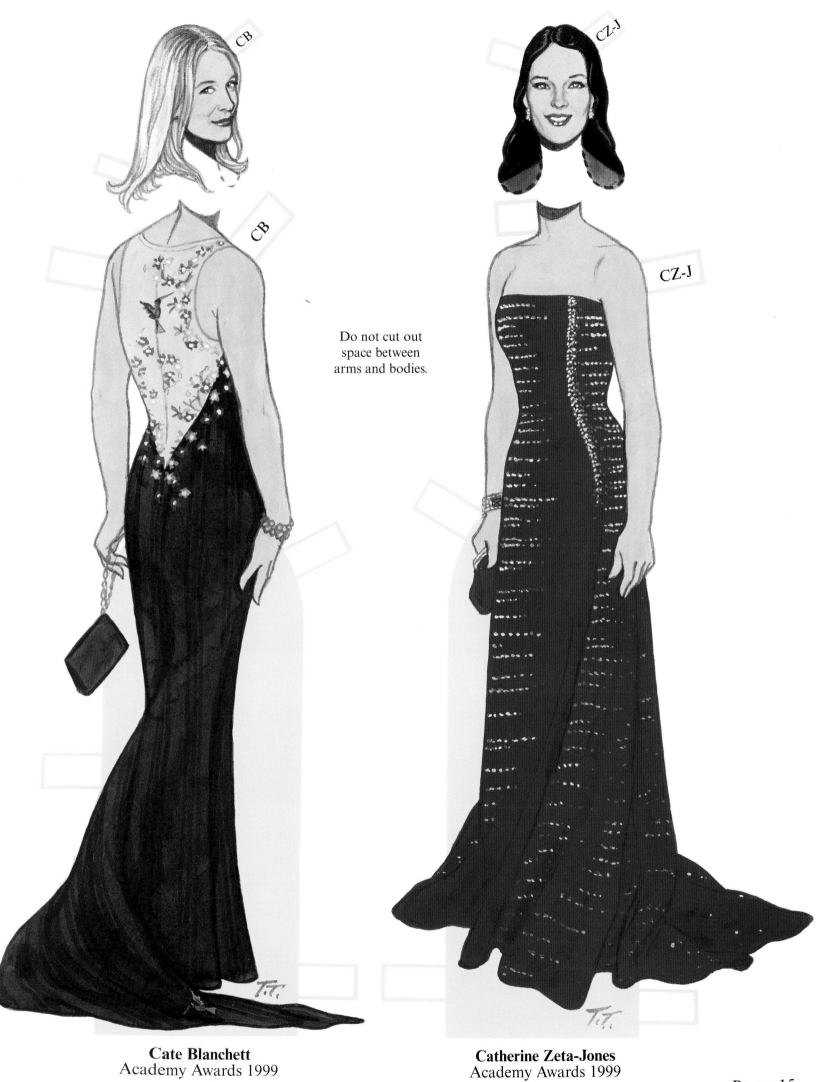

CB

CB

Do not cut out
space between
arms and bodies.

CZ-J

CZ-J

Cate Blanchett
Academy Awards 1999

Catherine Zeta-Jones
Academy Awards 1999

PLATE 15

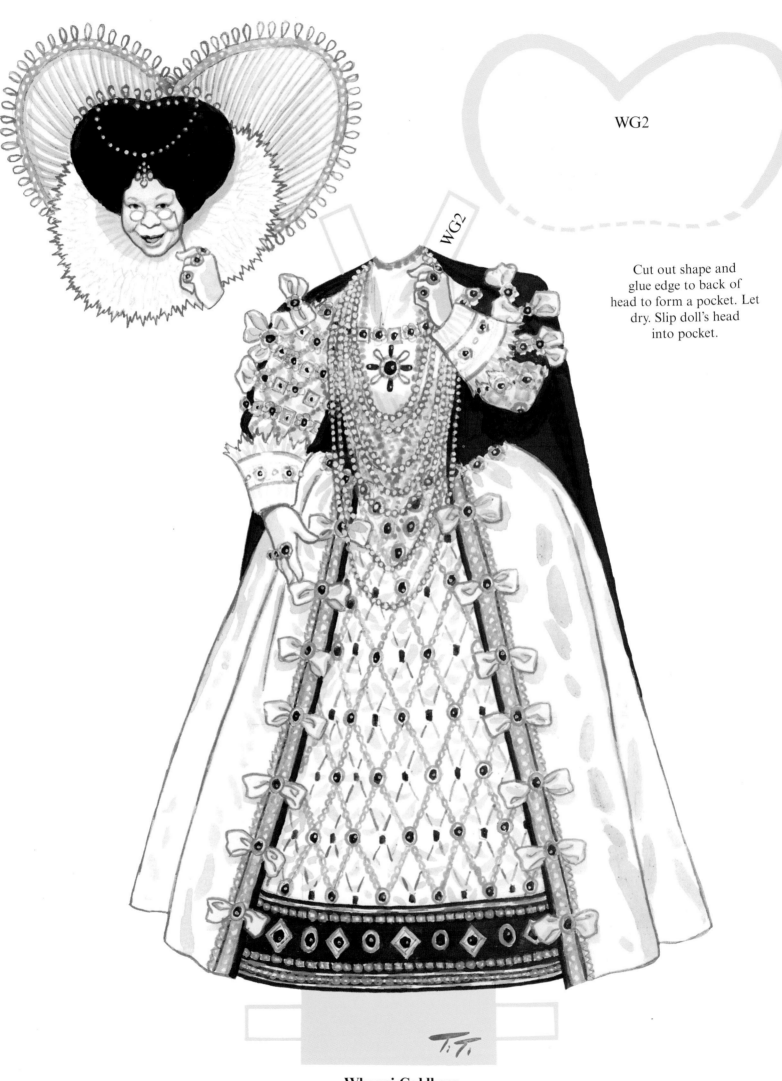

WG2

Cut out shape and
glue edge to back of
head to form a pocket. Let
dry. Slip doll's head
into pocket.

WG2

Whoopi Goldberg
Academy Awards 1999

PLATE 16